Yes, You're Fat!

I Like You Anyway

Straight-Forward Advice, Opinions, Truths and No Holds Barred Stuff to keep you on the path to being Skinny!

Warning: Not for the overly sensitive

Rich DiGirolamo

Yes, You're Fat! I Like You Anyway!
Copyright © 2016 by Rich DiGirolamo
Second Edition

Rich DiGirolamo

www.richdigirolamo.com

-1-

You will not lose weight every week while dieting. Stop reading this book right now if you think otherwise and give it to someone who is in touch with reality.

-2-

You are one smart cookie! You're still reading. Chances are you've probably eaten one too many cookies too!

-3-

And speaking of cookies, your kids do not *need* cookies. No one does.

-4-

Stop drinking soda. It is loaded with sugar and will give you cavities.

-5-

Keep a journal of what you eat.

-6-

Take a fifteen minute walk daily.
Look in people's windows.

-7-

Try a new vegetable today. The
worst thing that can happen is you
bite into it and find out you needed
to remove the skin.

-8-

"WE only THINK we're not worth it. But what do WE know?"
– Michelle Gotay

-9-

Do not eat fast food if possible. It clogs arteries and offers you the opportunity to Super-Size your clothes.

-10-

Be persistent with your actions.

-11-

Be consistent with your exercise.

-12-

Buy flattering clothes.
You deserve them.

-13-

Play with your food.

-14-

Being Skinny is a state of mind.
Relocate there!
It might not be warm and sunny,
but it will help you look hot!

-15-
Buy that bikini.

-16-
You're never too fat to ride a bicycle.

-17-
Stop weighing yourself every day. It gives you false hope and allows you to do dumb things.

-18-

Make your food fun.

-19-

Quit buying elastic pants. They
make you look even bigger than you
already are.

-20-

Stop wearing black. You're not
dead. But if you keep eating the
way you have been…………..

-21-

Go OUT for ice cream. Make it a family event.

-22-

Find a support mechanism and use it often.

-23-

Do not make enough for leftovers. Most leftovers remain in the refrigerator and end up turning into something scary looking.

-24-

Cut back on your sugar.

-25-

Cook!

-26-

Bring your lunch to work tomorrow. And when you're done eating take a co-worker out for a walk. A leash is optional.

-27-

Stop offering others advice and start using it yourself.

-28-

Quit making excuses. Too many "Buts" have led to your huge Butt!

-29-

Write a list of all the things you will do when you're Skinny. Let the sky be the limit.

-30-

Eat a healthy dessert every day.

-31-

Be the first to order at the restaurant and make the better choice.

-32-

Start a Volleyball game at a picnic. This might require you bringing a ball and a net. (You were going to bring cookies, weren't you?)

-33-

Drink water.

-34-

Take another walk.

-35-

Shop a health food store every so often.

-36-

Join or visit a food co-op.

-37-

Plan a great outing when you reach your goal.

-38-

Visit an outdoor produce market.

-39-

It's 10:00 PM. How many times have you weighed yourself today?

Rich DiGirolamo

-40-

You did not buy it for your spouse or your kids. You're not that nice. You bought it for you! And you don't need it. Your butt is getting bigger.

-41-

Buy a smaller size. Try it on regularly until it fits. Every January is not regularly.

-42-

Monday is the wrong day to start dieting. Today is the right day.

-43-

Find skinny friends. Spend less time with fat friends. All they like to do is eat.

-44-

You do not need candy.

-45-

Buy a new cookbook. Use it. Make a commitment to try one new recipe every week.

-46-

Teach your family to cook.

-47-

Think Thin.

-48-

"Quit Looking For Reasons You Can't Accomplish Something"
– Rich DiGirolamo

-49-
Go outside and play.

-50-
You're not hungry. Most people reading this book have no idea what hunger is. Go visit a third world country; you'll learn about hunger.

-51-
Get up fifteen minutes earlier tomorrow and move your butt.

-52-
Have a snowball fight.

-53-
Have a water gun fight.

-54-
Stop baking cookies.
They make you fat.

-55-
If you must bake, have one!
Not one dozen.

-56-

Pat yourself on the back when you overcome a food challenge.

-57-

And when those annoying people start to make those comments......... Tell them to mind their own weight.

-58-

Dream small. Then dream big!

-59-
Buy sexy lingerie.

-60-
Corn chips smell like a dog's paws.

-61-
Do not take weight loss advice from an overweight doctor.

-62-
Wear that sexy lingerie.

-63-

There is no quick fix to losing weight. Period. End of discussion.

-64-

Prescription diet pills kill people!

-65-

Losing weight is not easy.
Accept it.

-66-

Losing weight sucks. But the rewards are awesome.

-67-

Stop eating bran turds.

-68-

Grill fruits and vegetables.

-69-

Dance your butt off!

-70-

Yes, you do look fat in that outfit. Now do something about it. Buying a larger size is not doing something about it.

-71-

You are not trying hard enough. And you know it.

-72-

Quit resisting change. Some day you will look back and ask yourself why you waited so long.

-73-

Do you want to be dead before your kids get married?

-74-

Do you want to see your grandchildren?

-75-

You should not lose 30 lbs. in 30 days. It is not safe. It is not healthy. It is just plain dumb. So stop calling those phone numbers you see plastered on telephone poles.

-76-

You have a cute butt.

-77-

Jump in a pile of leaves.

-78-

Yes, that heart attack can happen to YOU! How much longer are you going to play with fire?

-79-
Throw out the candy.

-80-
Throw out the cookies.

-81-
Throw out all the tempting crap.

-82-
Better yet. Stop buying it already
if you want to keep your cute butt.

-83-
Walk a little further.

-84-
Eat your lunch in a park.

-85-
Take the stairs, not the elevator.

-86-

Yes, you're fat.
I like you anyway!

I like your smile, your personality, and your morals, values and ethics, just to name a few things.

-87-

Buy that provocative outfit. Wear it proudly.

-88-

It was only five lbs. five lbs. ago. Should we shoot for fifteen?

-89-

The clothes dryer does not shrink zippers.

-90-

You're not overweight, you're under-tall. There are not many ways to get taller. They involve torture. So lose weight.

-91-

Be the cool, hip adult. Play with the kids in the neighborhood.

-92-

Never food shop when you are hungry.

-93-

Do not shop for groceries with children.

-94-

Learn the following words: small, few, less, one, mini, half, appetizer portion.

-95-

Learn the following response: "No, thank you. I am satisfied and it was delicious"

-96-

For the mommies: There is such thing as half a sandwich and you can always make another half.

-97-

Items offering "33% more free" have done nothing but increase your physical size by 33%.

-98-

Did you ever notice Buy 1 Get 2 Free sales do not involve lettuce?

-99-

Go out for a cup of coffee. Coffee.
Not coffee and…….

-100-

Don't lie. Your stomach will grow.

-101-

Find the end of a rainbow.

-102-

Drink milk. It builds strong bones.

-103-

Carbohydrates are not bad.
Eating too much of anything is bad.

-104-

Stop planning your day around food.

-105-

Keep a record of your weight loss.

-106-

Join a gym. Visit it after you join.

-107-

Have more sex. Take note of duration and stamina with each encounter.

-108-

Go catch a sunset.

-109-

Stop visiting buffets. The person before you picked their nose.

-110-

Traces of urine have been found on those after-dinner mints as you leave a restaurant.

-111-

Yes, you can be thin.

-112-

Being thin requires hard work. Hard work is something most people hate.

-113-

Wear something spandex.

-114-
Plan your meals.

-115-
People who lose weight cannot sit on hard chairs for very long. And you always wondered why pillows were invented.

-116
Tell them you can help them; just not now. Now go make yourself a healthy dinner.

-117

Stop saying you want to lose weight and actually do it already.

-118-

Stop whining about how fat you are. No one cares.

-119-

Buy things that support your weight loss efforts – no matter what the price. You have wasted too much money not doing this.

-120-

You "LOSE" weight. You do not "LOOSE" weight. Learn how to spell.

(Note: this one really irritates me!! Especially when people in the field of weight loss get it wrong. Morons!)

-121-

Stop trying to lose weight every January. Lose it now.

-122-

It is okay to lose $\frac{1}{2}$ lb per week.

-123-

No, you do not have it under control. Stop telling us that to avoid the conversation.

-124-

Yes, you know what you have to do to lose weight. But can you tell me why you are still not doing it?

-125-

You did not cheat on your diet. Look at it as a learning experience.

-126-

Listen to great speakers talk about weight loss success.

-127-

Yes, men lose weight faster.
Get over it.

-128-

Your spouse will still be a moron
long after you have devoured the
box of cookies.

-129-

You had your period last week.
Maybe even the week before.
Throw out the chocolate already.

-130-

You will not exercise every day until you die.

-131-

And this twice per day nonsense? Get real!

-132-

Eat five servings of fruits and vegetables every day. Candy corn is not a vegetable.

-133-

Why is it that you will throw out vegetables that have gone bad, but you never seem to throw out a cake that has gone bad?

-134-

There is always another option. Please do not forget that.

-135-

If you eat it, the starving children won't get it anyway. So throw it out, you've had enough.

-136-

There is no such club as The Clean Plate Club. But perhaps you can start The Huge Butt Club.

-137-

Read books about weight loss success.

-138-

Try two meals per day while vacationing. They should not last three hours each.

-139-

Put this book in your bathroom. Read it while doing your business.

-140-

Read this book over and over again. When you can recite it from memory you will be Skinny!

-141-

Find a proven weight loss program and follow it.

-142-

The right time to lose weight is now.

-143-

What's for dinner tonight?

-144-

There is a good possibility you will often be cold after you lose your weight. Start sweater shopping now. Smaller size please.

-145-

Don't you think one was enough?

-146-

ASK is one of the most powerful three letter words in the English language. Ask for your meals to be prepared your way.

-147-

You do not have the body of an eighteen year old. You probably never will again.

-148-

When was the last time you picked your own produce in a field?

-149-

Changes need to be permanent. Stop making drastic, unrealistic changes that will not last. But more importantly, stop trying to convince yourself that those drastic, unrealistic changes will last.

-150-

Play with people thinner than you. Learn from their actions.

-151-

Take half your meal home from the restaurant. You won't have to cook tomorrow.

-152-

You did not get fat eating too many vegetables. Stop asking if there is such a thing as too many vegetables.

-153-

You were a size two at birth.
It is time to grow up.

-154-

Yes, you were Skinny when you
smoked. You also smelled like a
cesspool. We are glad you stopped
smoking. Now suck up, stop eating
and try some exercise.

-155-

Order a child's portion. It is okay.
You won't starve.

-156-

Glistening vegetables are usually not fat-free.

-157-

Do not revolve your life around a scale.

-158-

Pasta is not bad for you; unless you eat it by the pound.

-159-

Plant a vegetable garden.

-160-

Broiled often means in fat or in butter. Ask. There is that word again.

-161-

Get rid of the goody cabinet. Downsize to a shelf or drawer and you will watch yourself down a size or two.

-162-

You are the mommy. Enough said.

-163-

Food will not bring back a dead
loved one.

-164-

Humpty Dumpty was scraped off
the floor and scrambled up with
some onions, peppers, mushrooms
and salsa. Try it.

-165-

Help others lose weight. Everyone
has tips and tricks that work.
Even you. Share them.

-166-

Ask for help when it is needed.
Others have ideas that just might
help you. People want to help you.
But please do not chew them up and
spit them out when they tell you
that which you do not wish to hear.

-167-

Hang around with people larger than
you. It is good for your ego.

-168-

When all else fails, opt for surgery
I said ALL ELSE.

-169-

It is not about willpower. It is
about how bad you want to be
thinner.

-170-

How do you know you're hungry? I
do not see you passed out on the
floor.

-171-

Plant an herb garden. Cook with fresh herbs on a regular basis. Do not plant "that" herb.

-172-

Reward yourself often.

-173-

Stop putting everyone else's needs first. Take care of you. Tell them you <u>can</u> help them; but offer a time that works for you.

-174-

Put time in the family schedule for you.

-175-

Take your lunch to the beach.

-176-

Yes, your face is pretty. So what!

-177-

What number attempt is this at losing weight? What year is it?

-178-

What is really eating at you?

-179-

Cry. Scream. Laugh. Let the emotion run its course instead of you running to the cupboard.

-180-

Tell people how hard you are working at losing weight.

-181-

It is not a diet. It is personal development. Personal development is a process that takes time, dedication and looking hard at oneself.

-182-

Men will not put the seat down. Women won't leave it up. Let's call it a draw.

-183-

Fat-free does not mean calorie free. Some of you still have not figured that one out. You are making the fat free industry very rich. They send their thanks.

-184-

"Do or Do not.
There is No Try"
- Yoda

-185-

As far as I am
concerned there is no
Do Not. Now go Do.

-186-

In the game of weight loss, it is okay to be a loser.

-187-

A snow day should not mean bake cookies. Go outside and make a ~~snowman~~ person

-188-

Eat Marshmallow Peeps. They're delicious!

-189-

Beans, beans, good for your heart, the more you eat the more weight you'll lose.

-190-

Throw out your fat clothes. If you keep them, you *WILL* need them again. This one is not optional. Do it now. If you don't, you're stupid.

-191-

Eating healthier does not cost more when you factor in fewer co-pays.

-192-

Fad diets do not work.

-193-

Trust the process of losing weight.

-194-

Goodwill and Salvation Army stores can be great places to shop for interim sizes while losing.

-195-

Involve others in your weight loss. Most people cannot do this alone.

-196-

All-You-Can-Eat is one reason you now own this book. Stop searching out those places.

-197-

Toss Brussels sprouts in a small amount of olive oil and seasonings. Bake until they are black. They are delicious. Thanks Beth!

-198-

Stop by a roadside fruit stand. Buy a piece of fruit instead of stopping somewhere for a candy bar.

-199-

"It is not that you do not like a food; you haven't found a way that you like it" – Brandi Hayden

-200-

Yes, people are noticing how much food you eat. Yes, they are talking about you! Yes, they are not saying nice things.

-201-

Why are you always the first one to finish eating?

-202-

Use your outdoor grill year-round.

-203-

Did you get to the gym yet *THIS* week?

-204-

Stop saying bad things about your weight. You have me to abuse you.

-205-

Get a good set of measuring spoons and use them.

-206-

Stop reading all the conflicting information on diets. Pick the best information for you. This book should be considered standard reading for everyone you know involved in weight loss or weight management. Don't be cheap. Buy them one.

-207-

Keep a running list of every little success. Review it often.

-208-

Show your family where the kitchen is located when they start complaining about your healthier meals.

-209-

A bag of microwave popcorn is not dinner. Stop being lazy!

-210-

Stop eyeing the last piece. You do not need it. You have had enough.

-211-

Healthy choices are available at a Chinese restaurant.

-212-

Stop thinking exercise is a license to eat.

-213-

Yes, you actually can buy one piece of cake at a bakery.

-214-

You have no intention of giving up sweets forever. Stop saying you will. So let's get a handle on them once and for all.

-215-

You do not love vegetables and you know it. So stop saying it already. They are good for you. They provide basic nutrition. But love?

-216-

It is normal to binge every so often. I said every so often.

-217-

Let someone else have the biggest slice of pizza. You already have the biggest something else.

-218-

Why do you eat healthy meals yet you continue to let your loved ones fill their bodies with crap?

-219-

Try one new vegetable every week.

-220-

Get rid of the size four already. It probably is doing more harm than good hanging in your closet.

-221-

Choose a smart weight goal; one that you can maintain.

-222-

Those people on those exercise equipment infomercials did not get those bodies in
twenty minutes. They probably did not even get those bodies on those machines.
You won't either.

-223-

Take your can for a walk. Grab two cans of soup and add some resistance as you go strolling through the neighborhood.

-224-

Go drink another glass of water right now.

-225-

Stop hiding behind sweaters and coats. It makes coping much easier when spring and summer arrive.

-226-

Try climbing the steps to get to your twelve-step meeting.

-227-

Do not buy any sugary or fat-laden snacks on your next grocery store visit. You will be surprised how fruit can satisfy that evening urge.

-228-

Please stop wearing that blouse where the buttons are practically popping off. We really do not care to look at your bra.

-229-

People should like you for who you are, not what you look like.

-230-

If they like you better now that you are skinny, tell them to take a hike.

-231-

Please do not date anyone who was not hot for you before you lost weight. Have some pride!

-232-

Do not ever cook two meals. They eat what you cook or hand them a box of cereal.

-233-

Take an exercise class with a friend.

-234-

Each morning write five things you will accomplish today on your weight loss journey.

-235-

Stop dressing Dumpy and Frumpy.

-236-

Tap water is free.

-237-

You could gain five pounds in the next forty-eight hours. Care to try?

-238-

I just love the food stains on your clothes. They tell me a lot about your eating habits.

-239-

Shop for clothes in a consignment store. Great deals are abundant.

-240-

Never wear stretch pants to a holiday dinner.

-241-

Come to think of it, never wear stretch pants. They make you look fatter.

-242-

When vacationing, shop for clothes and jewelry, not salt water taffy.

-243-

When mom is happy, everyone is happy.

-244-

What do you mean there's nothing in this house to eat? Shop for groceries on a regular basis.

-245-

Buy a crock pot. Now you have no excuse not to eat a healthy meal.

-246-
Eat breakfast.

-247-
"You THINK you're a closet eater? Just remember you're not alone in that closet. Your thighs are spies."
- Rosemary Chiaverini

-248-
"I only eat one meal a day. Why am I fat?" Read again.

-249-

Fat people are not jolly.
They are miserable.

-250-

Fat people are not jolly.
They are uncomfortable.

-251-

Fat people are not jolly.
They are just like everyone
else – flesh and blood; with
feelings and emotions.

-252-

Learn the difference between a tablespoon and a ladle.

-253-

Stop buying Halloween candy in August. You will end up buying it again. Buy it two days before or you deserve to get fat.

-254-

Buy yourself flowers. Keep them near you while you cook.

-255-

Place a huge bowl of fruit on your counter. Fill it weekly.

-256-

Rent a bicycle when you are in a new city. You will see more sights.

-257-

Do some form of daily exercise.

-258-

How many different varieties of lettuce have you eaten?

-259-

How about varieties of ice cream?

-260-

Choose a weight goal that is not based on vanity.

-261-

Try vegetarianism for one week. Deer do it and look how cute they are.

-262-

Everyone has personal issues. Yours are just noticeable. For now!

-263-

Your skinny, rich, beautiful friend's husband is cheating on her.

-264-

Some people still feel fat even after losing a lot of weight.

-265-

I heard you ask when this will be over. It is never over.

-266-

And why didn't you keep it off the last time? And are you going to take the same approach again?

-267-

Fat-free cheese is not a food.

-268-

Buy a food scale. Use it.

-269-

Ice cream and frozen yogurt are not milk products.

-270-

The following items can be found at a buffet:

Bacteria

Urine

Feces

Fungus

E.coli

Trash

Bon Appetit!

-271-

Eat right. Set a good example for your kids. You can screw them up in other areas.

-272-

I am glad you have a treadmill. It is quite obvious you are not using it.

-273-

Ever wonder why they are sabotaging you? How many times have you told them you're going to lose weight?

-274-

Some people will not like you when you lose weight. Their loss.

-275-

On your next vacation, rent a house or condo instead of a hotel room. Cook and keep fresh fruits and veggies around for snacking. Then dine out and indulge a couple of times. You'll feel in control.

-276-

Plan a vacation with people who like to do things other than eat.

-277-

Do not use your car one day each week. Use your legs to get around.

-278-

Position yourself away from the food at parties.

-279-

Veggie burgers are pre-cooked. You need to heat them up. Stop waiting for flames to shoot up from the BBQ. That is why you think they suck.

-280-

Tell your spouse/partner/significant other that they are cut off if they bring home candy for Valentine's Day.

-281-

You can lose weight during menopause. It may not be easy, but it can be done.

-282-

You do not need motivation. Everyone is motivated. What you need to figure out is what motivates you to succeed.

-283-

The phrase "Lifestyle Change" is overrated.

-284-

The phrase "Lifestyle Change" is overused.

-285-

Change your life, not your lifestyle.

-286-

Most people have cookie ingredients in their home at any given time. A lot of good that does.

-287-

Do not lose weight for a reunion. You will just gain it all back.

-288-

Get a new haircut. Just changing your appearance can make you feel thinner.

-289-

Thin people work the room at a party. Fat people work at refilling serving plates.

-290-

When I was eighteen years old, my thirty-six year old neighbor died from overdosing on over-the-counter appetite suppressants.

-291-

Buy fruit that is already cut up. It costs about the same as that nasty, greasy fast food meal.

-292-

Have a well stocked pantry.

-293-

Do not drive to the bottom of your driveway to pick up your mail. You make it much too easy for people to comment about your size.

-294-

Muscle does weigh more than fat. You did not build up that much muscle this week. So tell me again why you did not lose weight?

-295-

Carry a water bottle wherever you go. Fill it before you head out. Bring it home empty.

-296-

Keep your kitchen clean. Who wants to cook or eat in a messy kitchen?

-297-

Believe in yourself. I believe in you.

Rich DiGirolamo

-298-

Believe your efforts will be
rewarded. Of course, you might
need to help with the reward
process.

-299-

Gather brochures of clothing that
you have only dreamed about
wearing.

-300-

Don't eat and drive.

-301-

If this was easy, everyone would be a supermodel.

-302-

Even thin people struggle with weight issues. Go ahead and ask them.

-303-

Man cannot live on salad alone.

-304-

This week you are going to do it. You told me that last week too! Or maybe I should be asking you what "IT" is?

-305-

The opinions of overweight people do matter. And if you think not, read this again.

-306-

No, you should not have another one. You already can't see your toes.

-307-
Take human bites

-308-
Join an outdoor club. Take up walking or hiking.

-309-
They do make nice clothing in larger sizes. Buy some.

-310-
Most models are anorexic.

-311-

Blame it on your children. They ruined your figure. Remind them of this when they want you to miss your exercise class.

-312-

Save money. Drink water at a restaurant.

-313-

Share a dessert with a loved one. It will ensure that you will still be able to share the same bed.

-314-

It is only food. It is in abundance. Please refrain from thinking you will never see it again.

-315-

The first bite usually tastes best.

-316-

The second bite does not taste as good as the first bite.

-317-

The third bite is where guilt, shame and disgust start to kick in.

-318-

The fourth bite sucks!

-319-

You are what you eat. Too bad some of you are nothing but sugar and lard.

-320-

Stop telling us you will lose weight. Just shut up and do it already.

-321-

Could you have a tag sale solely devoted to exercise equipment you bought and were going to use?

-322-

Laugh at your mistakes. But learn from them too!

-323-

Stuff a tomato!

-324-

"You can have your cake and eat it too; just not on the same day" – Linda Wilkinson

-325-

Have some fun – every day.

-326-

The real question is "Are you READY to lose weight?"

-327-

Ten minutes not sitting on the sofa with a bag of chips between your legs is a good thing. Go shake your groove thing.

-328-

Take a cooking class.

-329-

Watching TV will not make you skinny.

-330-

You did not just wake up one day to find yourself fat. It took years of grooming. It will take some time to lose it as well.

-331-

Smart people do not offer to help. So ask if you need help.

-332-

You seem to have all the answers about losing weight. So why are you still fat?

-333-

Do not tell us you have no time to do things for yourself. How many times did you hit snooze this morning?

-334-

The Problem is…………..
YOU!

-335-

It is really possible to lose weight permanently and keep it off.

How?

Read my final thought.

-336-

Take heed to all the stuff you have just read. Use it and take it to heart. Or else you are destined to a fat, unhappy, unhealthy life.

Now, Go Get Skinny!

Disclaimer: Injury, illness, hurt feelings, or death from reading this book is not my problem. I free myself of any responsibility.

For information regarding quantity purchases of this book, personal development workshops, coaching or other speaking services contact:

Rich DiGirolamo

rich@richdigirolamo.com
Visit www.richdigirolamo.com